THE COMPLETE GOLO DIET COOKBOOK FOR BEGINNERS 2024

Quick Flavorful Healthy Recipes to Reduce Inflammation, Sustainable Weight Loss, Improved Insulin Sensitivity and Overall Health

Dr. Raphael Rachelle

TABLE OF CONTENTS

ENCOURAGEMENT

Embarking on the Golo Diet or any lifestyle change can be both exciting and challenging. Here are some words of encouragement to support you on this journey:

Start with Purpose

Embrace Your Why: Remind yourself why you've chosen this path. Whether it's improved health, more energy, or weight management, let that purpose be your driving force.

Patience and Progress

Embrace Progress: Every small step counts. Acknowledge and celebrate each achievement, no matter how minor it may seem.

Patience is Key: Lifestyle changes take time. Be patient with yourself and the process. Results will come with consistency and perseverance.

Positive Mindset

Mind over Matter: Your mindset is a powerful tool. Stay positive and believe in your ability to make positive changes in your life.

Shift Focus: Instead of fixating on what you can't eat, concentrate on the delicious and nutritious foods you can enjoy.

Self-Compassion

Be Kind to Yourself: Recognize that setbacks are an inevitable part of the process. Show yourself compassion and treat yourself with kindness during challenging times.

Support and Community

Community and Support: Seek guidance and support from friends, family, or online communities. Sharing experiences and receiving encouragement can be invaluable.

Accountability Partner: Consider having someone to share your journey with. An accountability partner can offer motivation and help keep you on track.

Education and Adaptation

Stay Informed: Knowledge is power. Educate yourself about the principles of the Golo Diet and why it works. Stay open to learning and adapting your approach as needed.

Consistency

Small Steps Daily: Consistency in making small, healthier choices every day adds up to significant changes over time.

Every Effort Counts: Even if a day doesn't go as planned, each effort towards your goal is a step forward. Keep moving forward!

Celebrate Achievements

Celebrate Victories: Celebrate every milestone, whether it's trying a new recipe, feeling more energetic, or sticking to your plan for a week. Every achievement is a step closer to your objective.

Remember, you are taking an important step towards a healthier and happier you. Embrace the journey, stay determined, and be proud of yourself for committing to a positive change. You're making an investment in your well-being, and that's truly something to be celebrated!

INTRODUCTION

In the heart of the vibrant city of New York, Sarah found herself at a crossroads. Struggling with weight management and feeling the strains of a hectic urban lifestyle, she was on a quest for a sustainable solution that wouldn't just help her shed pounds but would also prioritize her overall well-being.

Amidst the bustling cityscape and the hustle of her daily routine, Sarah stumbled upon "The Complete Golo Diet Cookbook for Beginners." Drawn in by the promises of a diet that emphasized not just weight loss, but also stable insulin levels and improved health, she decided to give it a try.

Armed with the vibrant pages of this cookbook, Sarah embarked on a journey that transformed her relationship with food and her health. The book wasn't just a compilation of recipes; it was a beacon of guidance, providing her with a roadmap to navigate the complex landscape of urban living while still prioritizing her health.

As she dove into the colorful recipes and practical meal plans, Sarah discovered a newfound joy in the kitchen. No longer was cooking a chore; it became an adventure, exploring a myriad of nutrient-dense, flavorful dishes that satisfied her taste buds while aligning with the principles of the Golo Diet.

With time, Sarah noticed remarkable changes not only in her weight but also in her energy levels and overall well-being. She felt empowered, taking charge of her health through a diet that was both effective and sustainable. Armed with the tools and knowledge from "The Complete Golo Diet Cookbook for Beginners," Sarah not only shed unwanted pounds but also embraced a lifestyle that resonated with her - one that was balanced, delicious, and, most importantly, fulfilling.

Today, Sarah stands tall as a testament to the success of the Golo Diet. Her journey from confusion to clarity, from struggling to thriving, serves as an inspiration for countless others seeking a holistic and effective approach to health and weight management. The book wasn't just a guide; it was a game-changer that unlocked a world of possibilities for Sarah, an American who reclaimed her vitality and well-being with the help of the Golo Diet.

Brief overview of the Golo Diet principles

The Golo Diet is a weight loss program designed to manage insulin levels to promote weight loss and overall health. The core principles of the Golo Diet are centered on maintaining stable blood sugar levels and optimizing insulin responses.

Insulin Management: Focuses on controlling insulin levels to aid in weight loss. The program emphasizes the significance of maintaining balanced blood sugar and insulin for overall health and sustainable weight management.

Whole Foods Emphasis: Encourages the consumption of nutrient-dense, whole foods such as vegetables, lean proteins, and complex carbohydrates to help regulate blood sugar levels.

Avoidance of Processed Foods: Discourages highly processed and refined foods that can cause spikes in blood sugar levels, leading to increased insulin production.

Metabolic Support: Utilizes a natural supplement known as Release, designed to support metabolic health by aiding in insulin regulation and potentially reducing cravings.

Balanced Meals: Advocates for well-balanced meals, including appropriate portions of proteins, fats, and carbohydrates, to keep insulin levels steady and promote satiety.

Regular Eating Patterns: Promotes consistent meal timings to avoid blood sugar fluctuations, providing stable energy levels throughout the day.

Exercise and Physical Activity: Encourages regular physical activity as a complementary component to the diet for better overall health and enhanced weight loss.

Benefits of the Golo Diet for beginners

Simple Approach: The Golo Diet provides a straightforward and easy-to-understand approach to weight management, making it accessible for beginners who might be new to dieting or healthy eating strategies.

Stable Blood Sugar Levels: By focusing on foods that have a low impact on blood sugar and insulin levels, the diet helps in maintaining stable energy levels throughout the day, reducing the likelihood of energy crashes or cravings.

Weight Loss Support: The Golo Diet is designed to assist in weight loss by managing insulin levels, potentially reducing fat storage and aiding in the breakdown of stored fat, which can be particularly encouraging for beginners looking to shed excess weight.

Reduced Cravings: The emphasis on whole, nutrient-dense foods and the use of the Golo Release supplement may help in reducing cravings and overeating, providing beginners with a more manageable path to controlling their food intake.

Improved Overall Health: Beyond weight loss, the diet's focus on whole foods, balanced meals, and stable insulin levels can contribute to improved overall health, potentially reducing the risk of certain chronic conditions associated with high insulin levels, such as type 2 diabetes.

Sustainable Lifestyle Changes: By encouraging balanced eating habits and regular meal timings, the Golo Diet aims to promote sustainable lifestyle changes rather than quick fixes, which can be beneficial for beginners looking for a long-term approach to health and weight management.

Complementary Exercise Regimen: While the focus is primarily on nutrition and insulin management, the Golo Diet also emphasizes the importance of regular physical activity, which can be a motivating factor for beginners looking to incorporate exercise into their routines.

Types of Food Recommended and Restricted

Foods Recommended:

Whole Foods: Emphasis on whole, unprocessed foods such as fruits, vegetables, whole grains, lean proteins, and healthy fats.

Low-Glycemic Index Foods: Foods that have a low impact on blood sugar levels, such as non-starchy vegetables, legumes, whole grains, and some fruits like berries.

Lean Proteins: Chicken, turkey, fish, tofu, legumes, and other sources of lean protein are encouraged.

Healthy Fats: Avocado, nuts, seeds, olive oil, and other sources of healthy fats are recommended.

Fiber-Rich Foods: Foods high in fiber, such as whole grains, legumes, fruits, and vegetables, are promoted for their ability to regulate blood sugar.

Balanced Meals: Meals that include a balance of proteins, fats, and complex carbohydrates are encouraged to help maintain stable insulin levels.

Foods Restricted:

Highly Processed Foods: Highly processed and refined foods, including sugary snacks, white bread, pastries, and sugary drinks, should be limited or avoided.

High Glycemic Index Foods: Foods that can cause rapid spikes in blood sugar levels, such as white rice, white bread, sugary cereals, and candies, are restricted.

Excessive Starches: Limiting starchy foods like white potatoes and highly processed grains is recommended due to their impact on blood sugar.

Added Sugars: Sugary additives, such as table sugar, high-fructose corn syrup, and sweetened beverages, should be avoided.

Unhealthy Fats: Trans fats and excessive saturated fats, often found in fried foods and certain processed snacks, should be limited.

Processed Meats: Highly processed meats like sausages and certain deli meats with added sugars or unhealthy preservatives should be restricted.

How the Golo Diet supports weight loss and improved health

Insulin Management: By emphasizing foods that have a low impact on blood sugar levels, the Golo Diet helps regulate insulin, which can assist in reducing fat storage and promoting the breakdown of stored fat. This may lead to weight loss and the prevention of further weight gain.

Balanced Nutrition: The diet promotes a balanced intake of whole, nutrient-dense foods, including lean proteins, healthy fats, and complex carbohydrates, which can help maintain stable blood sugar levels. This balanced approach to nutrition supports overall health and energy levels.

Reduction in Cravings: By stabilizing blood sugar and insulin levels, the Golo Diet may reduce cravings and overeating, making it easier for individuals to manage their food intake and make healthier choices.

Whole Foods Emphasis: Emphasizing whole, unprocessed foods, the diet ensures a higher intake of essential nutrients, antioxidants, and fiber, supporting better overall health and reducing the risk of chronic diseases.

Physical Activity: The Golo Diet also encourages regular exercise, which not only supports weight loss but also contributes to improved cardiovascular health, increased metabolism, and enhanced overall well-being.

Supporting Metabolism: The Golo Diet incorporates the use of the Golo Release supplement, which aims to support metabolic health by assisting in insulin regulation, potentially reducing cravings, and supporting weight loss efforts.

Long-Term Approach: Rather than a quick-fix solution, the Golo Diet promotes sustainable lifestyle changes, encouraging a gradual and steady weight loss that is more likely to be maintained in the long term. This approach contributes to improved health over time.

Getting Started with the Golo Diet

Step-by-step guide for beginners

Understand the principles of the Golo Diet:

Learn about the Golo Diet's fundamental concepts, which include regulating insulin levels, promoting whole foods, and preparing balanced meals. Understand how diet affects blood sugar levels and insulin response.

Determine Your Health Goals:

Before you begin, evaluate your current health status, weight, and any existing medical concerns. Set realistic and defined objectives for your weight loss or health improvements with the Golo Diet.

Consult a Medical Professional:

Before beginning any new food plan, it's best to talk with a healthcare physician or a qualified dietitian, especially if you have any underlying health disorders or concerns.

Discover the Recommended Foods and Meal Structure:

Learn about the Golo Diet's suggested foods as well as those that should be limited or avoided. Understand the structure of balanced meals that include proteins, healthy fats, and complex carbohydrates.

Make a Meal Plan:

Create a meal plan based on the principles of the Golo Diet. Include complete foods, lean proteins, veggies, healthy fats, and carbohydrates with a low glycemic index in your meals.

Purchase Golo Diet Foods:

Shop for the recommended items and stock your pantry and fridge with them to ensure you have the right ingredients on hand to follow your meal plan.

Begin Recording Your Meals:

Keep a food journal or use a tracking app to log your meals, portions, and the effect on your energy levels. This might assist you in understanding how your body reacts to certain foods.

Include Exercise:

Begin or improve your workout program based on your ability and fitness level. The Golo Diet promotes regular physical activity as part of a comprehensive strategy to weight loss and improved health.

Introduce (if desired) Golo Release Supplement:

If you decide to use the Golo Release supplement, carefully follow the instructions and incorporate it into your daily routine as directed by the diet plan.

Maintain Consistency and Adaptability:

Maintain consistency in your meal plan, workout program, and supplements. Keep track of your progress, listen to your body, and be ready to change your strategy as needed for greater outcomes.

Introducing exercise and physical activity within the Golo Diet

Consult with a Healthcare Professional:

Before starting any exercise regimen, especially if you have pre-existing health conditions, consult a healthcare professional or a fitness expert to ensure the chosen activities align with your health status.

Choose Activities Suited to Your Fitness Level:

Select exercises that suit your current fitness level. This might include activities like brisk walking, cycling, swimming, or bodyweight exercises. Begin slowly and gradually raise the intensity as your fitness increases.

Aim for Regular Exercise:

Aim for a consistent exercise routine. The Golo Diet encourages at least 30 minutes of moderate exercise most days of the week. Find and keep to a schedule that's effective for you.

Combine Cardio and Strength Training:

Blend cardio exercises (like jogging, cycling, or dancing) with strength training (using weights, resistance bands, or bodyweight exercises).

This combination helps in burning calories, building muscle, and boosting metabolism.

Timing Your Exercise with Meals:

Consider timing your workouts strategically around your meals. For instance, exercising before a meal might assist in utilizing excess glucose in the bloodstream after eating, potentially managing blood sugar levels.

Stay Hydrated and Rested: Make sure you stay hydrated before, during, and after activity.

Ensure you're adequately hydrated before, during, and after exercise. Allow yourself proper rest and recovery time between workouts to prevent fatigue or overexertion.

Monitor Progress and Adapt:

Keep track of your fitness progress, such as increased endurance, strength, or weight loss. Adjust your exercise routine as needed to keep challenging your body and achieving your fitness goals.

Make Physical Activity a Habit:

Integrate physical activity into your daily routine. Take the stairs, walk or cycle for short distances, or find opportunities to move more throughout the day to supplement your structured workouts.

Enjoy the Process:

Find activities you enjoy. When you like the exercises you're doing, you're more likely to stick with them, making it a sustainable and enjoyable part of your lifestyle.

Recommended exercises and their benefits

Cardiovascular Workouts:

- Brisk walking or jogging: These activities raise the heart rate, which aids in the burning of calories and the improvement of cardiovascular health. They are easily accessible and adaptable to a variety of fitness levels.

- Cycling is a low-impact activity that helps to build leg muscles and burn calories. It can be done either outside or on a stationary bike.

- Dancing or Aerobics: Taking dance or aerobics courses is a fun way to burn calories, build endurance, and raise your heart rate.

- Swimming is a great cardiovascular exercise since it is a full-body workout that is easy on the joints.

Benefits:

Cardio exercises help to burn excess calories, boost metabolism, and improve heart and lung health. They aid in weight loss and blood sugar control.

Strengthening Exercises:

- Squats, lunges, push-ups, and planks are efficient bodyweight exercises for building muscle and strength.

- Resistance Training: Using resistance bands or weights to build muscle, increase metabolism, and maintain bone health is beneficial.

- Yoga or Pilates: These activities improve flexibility, core strength, and muscle tone, all of which contribute to overall fitness.

Benefits:

Strength training aids in the development and maintenance of muscle mass, which raises metabolism, improves insulin sensitivity, and aids in weight loss by burning more calories even when at rest.

HIIT (High-Intensity Interval Training):

- In HIIT, short bursts of intense exercise are followed by brief rest intervals. It can be applied to a variety of exercises, including cycling, running, and bodyweight training.

Benefits:

When compared to regular cardio activities, HIIT burns more calories, improves cardiovascular health, and boosts metabolism in less time.

Exercises for Flexibility and Mobility:

- Yoga and stretching: These exercises improve flexibility, alleviate muscle tension, and promote relaxation.

Benefits:

Flexibility exercises promote joint health, prevent injuries, and increase overall mobility and comfort during daily activities.

Tips for grocery shopping and pantry stocking

Grocery Shopping Tips:

- **Plan Ahead:** Create a detailed shopping list before heading to the store. This helps in buying only what's necessary and avoids impulse purchases.

- **Focus on Whole Foods:** Prioritize fresh produce, lean proteins, healthy fats, and whole grains. Opt for items with minimal processing and added sugars.

- **Read Labels:** Be mindful of food labels. Look for low-glycemic index options and choose items with lower added sugars and processed ingredients.

- **Stock Up on Vegetables:** Load up on a variety of non-starchy vegetables such as leafy greens, broccoli, bell peppers, and zucchini to use as the base for meals.

- **Choose Lean Proteins:** Select lean sources of protein like chicken, turkey, fish, tofu, legumes, and low-fat dairy products.

- **Include Healthy Fats:** Purchase sources of healthy fats like avocados, nuts, seeds, and olive oil for cooking and salad dressings.

Opt for Whole Grains: Pick whole grains such as quinoa, brown rice, whole-wheat pasta, and oats as healthier alternatives to refined grains.

Limit Processed Foods: Minimize highly processed items, sugary snacks, and beverages that can spike blood sugar levels.

Pantry Stocking Tips:

- **Whole Grain Options:** Stock whole-grain staples like brown rice, quinoa, whole-wheat flour, and oats for healthier carbohydrate choices.
- **Canned and Dried Goods:** Keep canned beans, lentils, and dried legumes for a convenient source of plant-based protein.
- **Healthy Cooking Oils:** Have olive oil, coconut oil, or avocado oil for healthier cooking and meal preparation.
- **Nuts and Seeds:** Store a variety of nuts (almonds, walnuts) and seeds (chia, flaxseed) for healthy snacking and to add to meals.
- **Herbs and Spices:** Keep a collection of herbs and spices to flavor meals without relying on excessive salt or high-calorie condiments.
- **Low-Sugar Snacks:** Have options like air-popped popcorn, dark chocolate, or fresh fruit available for healthier snack choices.
- Golo Diet Supplements (if using): If incorporating the Golo Release supplement, ensure it's part of your pantry stock and used as directed.

Essential kitchen tools and ingredients

Essential Kitchen Tools:

- **Quality Blender:** Useful for making smoothies, sauces, and soups using whole, nutritious ingredients.

- **Food Scale:** Helpful for portion control and accurate measurement of food items.

- **Non-Stick Pans or Skillets:** For cooking with minimal oil, especially when preparing lean proteins and vegetables.

- **Steamer Basket:** Ideal for steaming vegetables while retaining their nutrients.

- **Baking Sheets and Parchment Paper:** Useful for roasting vegetables or preparing healthier baked options.

- **Food Storage Containers:** For meal prepping and storing prepped ingredients or leftovers.

- **Sharp Knives and Cutting Boards:** Essential for cutting vegetables, fruits, and proteins.

- **Measuring Cups and Spoons:** Vital for precise measurement of ingredients for cooking and baking.

Common Ingredients for the Golo Diet:

- **Non-Starchy Vegetables:** Spinach, kale, broccoli, bell peppers, cauliflower, zucchini, and tomatoes.

- **Lean Proteins:** Chicken breast, turkey, fish (salmon, tuna), tofu, legumes (beans, lentils).

- **Healthy Fats:** Avocado, nuts (almonds, walnuts), seeds (chia, flaxseed), and olive oil.

- **Whole Grains:** Brown rice, quinoa, whole-wheat pasta, oats, and barley.

- Low-Glycemic Index Fruits: Berries (strawberries, blueberries, raspberries), apples, and citrus fruits.

- **Herbs and Spices:** Garlic, ginger, turmeric, basil, oregano, cinnamon, and others for flavoring without excessive use of salt or high-calorie condiments.

- **Low-Sodium Broth or Stock:** Vegetable or chicken broth for cooking and flavoring meals.

- **Golo Diet Supplement (if used):** The Golo Release supplement, as recommended by the diet plan.

- **Low-Sugar Dairy Alternatives:** Greek yogurt, unsweetened almond milk, and cheese with lower fat content.

- **Healthy Sweeteners:** Stevia or monk fruit sweetener for reducing sugar intake in recipes.

Breakfast Recipes

Berry and Greek Yogurt Parfait

Ingredients:

- 1 cup berries (strawberries, blueberries, and raspberries)
- 1 cup of Greek yogurt (unsweetened)
- 1/4 cup of granola (low-sugar or homemade)
- 1 tablespoon of chia seeds

Instructions:

- Add Greek yogurt, mixed berries, along with granola in a glass or bowl.
- Repeat the layering until all of the ingredients have been utilized.
- Top with a sprinkle of chia seeds for added fiber and omega-3s.
- Serve immediately for a nutritious and filling breakfast.

Veggie Omelette

Ingredients:

- 2 eggs
- 1/4 cup chopped red, green, or yellow bell peppers
- 1/4 cup chopped spinach
- 1/4 cup diced tomatoes
- 1 tablespoon olive oil

- Salt, pepper, and herbs to taste

Instructions:

- In a bowl, whisk the eggs and season with salt, pepper, and herbs.
- Warm the olive oil in a nonstick skillet over a medium-high heat.
- Add the diced vegetables and sauté until slightly tender.
- Pour the whisked eggs over the vegetables and cook until the omelette sets.
- Cook for a further minute after folding the omelette in half.
- Slide onto a plate and serve with a side of sliced avocado or whole-grain toast.

Overnight Chia Seed Pudding

Ingredients:

- 1/4 cup chia seeds
- 1 cup unsweetened almond milk or any preferred milk
- 1/2 teaspoon vanilla extract
- Berries or sliced fruits for topping

Instructions:

- In a jar or bowl, mix chia seeds, milk, and vanilla extract.
- Stir well and refrigerate overnight or for at least 4 hours until it thickens.
- In the morning, stir the pudding and add more milk if desired for consistency.
- Top with berries or sliced fruits before serving for a healthy and fiber-rich breakfast.

Nutritious and low-insulin-impact breakfast options

Veggie and Egg Scramble

Ingredients:

- 2 eggs
- 1/4 cup diced bell peppers
- 1/4 cup chopped spinach
- 1/4 cup diced tomatoes
- 1 tablespoon olive oil
- Spices and herbs (such as paprika, oregano, or thyme)
- Optional: 1/4 avocado (sliced)

Instructions:

- Warm the olive oil in a pan over a medium-low flame.
- Sauté the diced vegetables until slightly tender.
- Beat the eggs and add them to the pan with vegetables.
- Cook, stirring gently until the eggs are scrambled and fully cooked.
- Sprinkle with herbs and spices.
- Serve with a side of sliced avocado for healthy fats.

Greek Yogurt with Nuts and Berries

Ingredients:

- 1 cup Greek yogurt (unsweetened)
- 1/4 cup mixed nuts (almonds, walnuts)
- 1/4 cup mixed berries (blueberries, raspberries)
- Cinnamon for flavor

Instructions:

- In a bowl, add Greek yogurt.
- Top with mixed nuts and mixed berries.
- For extra taste, sprinkle with cinnamon.
- Mix together and enjoy this protein and fiber-rich breakfast.

Chia Seed Breakfast Bowl

Ingredients:

- 2 tablespoons chia seeds
- 1 cup unsweetened almond milk
- 1/4 cup sliced strawberries or other low-glycemic fruits
- 1 tablespoon unsweetened coconut flakes
- 1 tablespoon chopped nuts

Instructions:

- Chia seeds and almond milk should be combined in a bowl.

- Let it sit for 10 minutes, stirring occasionally until it thickens.

- Top the chia seed mixture with sliced strawberries, coconut flakes, and chopped nuts.

- Enjoy this high-fiber, low-sugar breakfast bowl.

Quinoa Breakfast Bowl

Ingredients:

- 1/2 cup cooked quinoa

- 1/4 cup unsweetened almond milk

- 1/4 cup diced apples

- 1 tablespoon chopped almonds

- Cinnamon for flavor

Instructions:

- In a bowl, combine cooked quinoa with almond milk.

- Add diced apples and chopped almonds.

- Sprinkle with cinnamon for added taste.

- Mix well and savor this protein and fiber-rich breakfast bowl.

Meal-prep ideas for busy mornings

Overnight Oats

Ingredients for One Serving:

- 1/2 cup rolled oats
- 1 cup unsweetened almond milk
- 1 tablespoon chia seeds
- 1/4 cup mixed berries (blueberries, strawberries)
- Cinnamon or vanilla extract for flavor

Instructions:

- In a mason jar or a bowl, combine rolled oats, almond milk, chia seeds, and your choice of flavoring (cinnamon or vanilla).
- Add mixed berries and mix well.
- Refrigerate the mixture overnight.
- In the morning, grab and enjoy your ready-to-eat breakfast.

Egg Muffins

Ingredients:

- 6 eggs
- 1/4 cup diced bell peppers
- 1/4 cup chopped spinach
- 1/4 cup diced tomatoes
- Salt, pepper, and herbs for seasoning

Instructions:

- Preheat the oven to 350°F (175°C).
- Whisk the eggs and season with salt, pepper, and herbs.
- Grease a muffin tin and distribute diced vegetables evenly into each cup.
- Pour the egg mixture over the vegetables.
- Bake for twenty to twenty-five minutes or until the egg muffins are firm.
- Once cooled, store them in an airtight container in the fridge. In the morning, microwave a quick breakfast.

Chia Seed Pudding Jars

Ingredients for One Serving:

- 2 tablespoons chia seeds
- 1 cup unsweetened almond milk
- Sliced fruits (e.g., kiwi, mango, or pineapple)
- Unsweetened coconut flakes

Instructions:

- In a jar, mix chia seeds and almond milk.
- Add your choice of sliced fruits and coconut flakes.
- Refrigerate overnight.
- In the morning, you have a convenient and nutritious chia seed pudding ready to grab and go.

Pre-Portioned Greek Yogurt Parfaits

Ingredients:

- Individual containers of Greek yogurt (unsweetened)
- Mixed nuts (almonds, walnuts)
- Sliced low-glycemic fruits (berries, apples)

Instructions:

- In individual containers, layer Greek yogurt, mixed nuts, and sliced fruits.
- Make a few portions and refrigerate for a quick breakfast option.

Lunch and dinner recipes

Quinoa Salad with Grilled Chicken

Ingredients:

- 1 cup cooked quinoa

- Grilled chicken breast (sliced)

- 1/4 cup cherry tomatoes (halved)

- 1/4 cup diced cucumber

- Mixed greens (spinach or arugula)

- Lemon vinaigrette, comprising of lemon juice, olive oil, salt, pepper

Instructions:

- In a bowl, mix cooked quinoa, mixed greens, cherry tomatoes, and diced cucumber.

- Add sliced grilled chicken on top.

- Toss gently with the lemon vinaigrette.

- Enjoy this protein-packed and filling salad.

Veggie Stir-Fry with Tofu

Ingredients:

- 1 block tofu (extra-firm, cubed)
- Stir-fry vegetables (bell peppers, broccoli, and snap peas)
- Low-sodium soy sauce or tamari
- Garlic, ginger, and sesame oil for seasoning
- Cooked brown rice or quinoa (optional)

Instructions:

- In a pan, heat sesame oil and stir-fry tofu until lightly browned. Set aside.
- In the same pan, stir-fry assorted vegetables with garlic and ginger until tender-crisp.
- Return the cooked tofu to the pan.
- Season with either tamari or low-sodium soy sauce.
- Serve alone or over a bed of brown rice or quinoa.

Baked Salmon with Steamed Vegetables

Ingredients:

- Salmon fillets
- Mixed vegetables (asparagus, carrots, broccoli)
- Lemon slices
- Olive oil, salt, and pepper
- Herbs (rosemary, thyme, or dill)

Instructions:

- Preheat the oven to 400°F (200°C).
- Season salmon with olive oil, salt, pepper, and herbs. Place lemon slices on top.
- Bake for twelve to fifteen minutes or till the salmon is done.
- Steam mixed vegetables and serve alongside the baked salmon.

Turkey Lettuce Wraps

Ingredients:

- Ground turkey
- Butter lettuce leaves
- Diced bell peppers and onions
- Low-sodium taco seasoning
- Avocado slices for topping

Instructions:

- In a pan, sauté ground turkey with diced vegetables and taco seasoning until cooked.
- Wash and separate the lettuce leaves for wrapping.
- Fill the lettuce leaves with the turkey mixture.
- Top with avocado slices and enjoy these low-carb wraps.

Balanced meal options for main courses

Grilled Lemon Herb Chicken with Roasted Vegetables

Ingredients:

- Chicken breasts or thighs
- Mixed vegetables (bell peppers, zucchini, red onion)
- Olive oil, lemon juice, garlic, herbs (rosemary, thyme)
- Salt and pepper to taste

Instructions:

- Marinate chicken with olive oil, lemon juice, garlic, and herbs for about 30 minutes.
- Preheat the grill. Grill the chicken until fully cooked.
- Mix the vegetables in a bowl along with the salt, pepper, and olive oil.
- Roast the vegetables in the oven until tender.
- Serve grilled chicken with roasted vegetables for a well-rounded meal.

Baked Tofu with Quinoa and Steamed Broccoli

Ingredients:

- Tofu (extra-firm, cubed)
- Quinoa (cooked)

- Broccoli florets

- Low-sodium soy sauce or tamari

- Olive oil, garlic, ginger

Instructions:

- Preheat the oven to 400°F (200°C).

- Toss tofu cubes with olive oil, garlic, and ginger.

- Bake tofu for 25-30 minutes until golden.

- Steam broccoli until tender-crisp.

- Serve baked tofu with cooked quinoa and steamed broccoli. Drizzle with low-sodium soy sauce or tamari for flavor.

Seared Salmon with Quinoa and Asparagus

Ingredients:

- Salmon fillets

- Quinoa (cooked)

- Fresh asparagus spears

- Lemon, olive oil, salt, and pepper

- Herbs (dill, parsley) for seasoning

Instructions:

- Season salmon with olive oil, salt, pepper, and herbs. Squeeze lemon juice on top.

- Sear the salmon in a pan until cooked to your liking.

- Steam or roast asparagus until tender.

- Serve seared salmon with a side of cooked quinoa and asparagus for a nutrient-rich meal.

Turkey and Vegetable Stir-Fry with Brown Rice

Ingredients:

- Ground turkey

- Vegetable stir-fry (bell peppers, snap peas, carrots)

- Low-sodium soy sauce or tamari

- Garlic, ginger, sesame oil

- Cooked brown rice

Instructions:

- Brown the ground turkey in a skillet.

- Stir-fry assorted vegetables with garlic, ginger, and sesame oil until tender-crisp.

- Combine cooked turkey and vegetables.

- Serve over a bed of brown rice, drizzled with low-sodium soy sauce or tamari.

Varieties of protein, vegetables, and healthy fats

Proteins:

Poultry:

- Chicken (breasts, thighs)
- Turkey (ground or whole)

Fish:

- Salmon
- Tuna
- Cod
- Trout

Plant-Based Proteins:

- Tofu
- Tempeh
- Lentils
- Chickpeas
- Black beans

Lean Meats:

- Beef cuts that are lean (such as sirloin or tenderloin)
- Pork tenderloin

Eggs:

- Whole eggs
- Egg whites

Vegetables:

Leafy Greens:

- Spinach
- Kale
- Swiss Chard

Cruciferous Vegetables:

- Broccoli
- Cauliflower
- Brussels sprouts

Colorful Vegetables:

- Bell peppers (red, green, yellow)
- Tomatoes
- Carrots

Root Vegetables:

- Sweet potatoes
- Beets
- Carrots

Others:

- Zucchini
- Asparagus
- Mushrooms

Healthy Fats:

Avocado:

- Rich in monounsaturated fats, great for salads, spreads, or as a snack.

Nuts:

- Almonds
- Walnuts
- Pistachios

Seeds:

- Chia seeds
- Flaxseeds
- Pumpkin seeds

Oils:

- Olive oil
- Avocado oil
- Coconut oil

Fatty Fish:

- Salmon
- Mackerel
- Sardines

Snacks and dessert recipes

Apple Sandwiches with Almond Butter

Ingredients:

- Apples (sliced crosswise)
- Almond butter (unsweetened)
- Optional toppings: Chia seeds, sliced almonds

Instructions:

- On a single apple slice, apply almond butter.
- To make a sandwich, top with another apple slice.
- Add chia seeds or sliced almonds for extra crunch and nutrients.
- Enjoy these nutritious and protein-rich apple sandwiches.

Veggie Sticks with Hummus

Ingredients:

- Vegetable sticks (carrots, cucumber, and bell peppers)
- Hummus (low-sodium)

Instructions:

- Wash and cut assorted vegetables into sticks.
- Serve with a side of hummus for a crunchy, fiber-rich snack.

Chia Seed Pudding with Berries

Ingredients:

- 3 tablespoons chia seeds
- 1 cup unsweetened almond milk
- Mixed berries (strawberries, blueberries, raspberries)
- Optional: Unsweetened coconut flakes

Instructions:

- Mix chia seeds and almond milk in a bowl. Refrigerate for at least 4 hours or overnight until it thickens.
- Layer chia seed pudding with mixed berries in a glass or bowl.
- Top with unsweetened coconut flakes for added texture and flavor.

Greek Yogurt with Honey and Nuts

Ingredients:

- Greek yogurt (unsweetened)
- Raw honey
- Mixed nuts (almonds, walnuts, pistachios)

Instructions:

- In a bowl, add Greek yogurt.
- Drizzle with raw honey for sweetness.
- Sprinkle mixed nuts on top for a crunchy and protein-rich dessert.

Dark Chocolate-Covered Berries

Ingredients:

- Dark chocolate (70% cocoa or higher)
- Mixed berries (strawberries, raspberries)

Instructions:

- In a heatproof bowl set over simmering water, melt dark chocolate.
- Dip the berries in the melted chocolate, ensuring they're coated.
- Place on a tray lined with parchment paper and let them cool until the chocolate hardens.

Satisfying and low-insulin-impact snack ideas

Cottage Cheese with Berries

Ingredients:

- Cottage cheese (low-fat or full-fat)
- Mixed berries (blueberries, strawberries, raspberries)

Instructions:

- Top a serving of cottage cheese with a handful of mixed berries for a high-protein and low-sugar snack.

Cucumber and Tuna Salad

Ingredients:

- Cucumber slices
- Canned tuna (in water)
- Olive oil, lemon juice, salt, pepper

Instructions:

- Mix drained tuna with olive oil, lemon juice, salt, and pepper. Spoon it onto cucumber slices for a refreshing, protein-rich snack.

Almond Butter and Celery Sticks

Ingredients:

- Celery sticks
- Almond butter (unsweetened)

Instructions:

- Fill celery sticks with almond butter for a satisfying, crunchy snack rich in healthy fats and fiber.

Hard-Boiled Eggs with Guacamole

Ingredients:

- Hard-boiled eggs
- Guacamole (homemade or store-bought)

Instructions:

- Cut hard-boiled eggs in half and top with guacamole for a protein and healthy fat-packed snack.

Greek Yogurt with Chia Seeds

Ingredients:

- Greek yogurt (unsweetened)
- Chia seeds

Instructions:

- Mix chia seeds into Greek yogurt for a low-sugar, high-protein snack that's rich in fiber and omega-3s.

Mixed Nuts and Seeds

Ingredients:

- Mixed nuts (almonds, walnuts, pistachios)
- Seeds (pumpkin seeds, sunflower seeds)

Instructions:

- Combine a handful of mixed nuts and seeds for a satisfying and nutrient-dense snack high in healthy fats and protein.

Veggie Stuffed Avocado

Ingredients:

- Avocado
- Diced vegetables (bell peppers, tomatoes, onions)
- Lemon juice, salt, pepper

Instructions:

- Scoop out some avocado and fill it with diced vegetables. Season with lemon juice, salt, and pepper for a filling and low-insulin-impact snack.

Healthier alternatives for sweet cravings

Fresh Fruit:

- **Berries:** Blueberries, strawberries, raspberries, and blackberries are lower in sugar compared to many other fruits.
- **Apples:** Satisfying and naturally sweet, apples can help curb sugar cravings.

Oranges: Rich in natural sugars and fiber, providing a sweet and tangy snack.

Dark Chocolate:

- Select dark chocolate with a higher cocoa percentage (70% or more) which tends to be lower in added sugars and higher in antioxidants. Enjoy a small piece or two to satisfy sweet cravings.

Greek Yogurt Parfait:

- Combine unsweetened Greek yogurt with fresh berries, a drizzle of honey or a small amount of granola for a balanced and slightly sweet treat.

Homemade Energy Balls:

- Prepare energy balls using ingredients such as dates, nuts, and a touch of unsweetened coconut flakes or cocoa powder. These provide a natural sweetness without added sugars.

Frozen Fruit:

- Freeze grapes, bananas, or berries for a refreshing and sweet frozen treat.

Chia Seed Pudding:

- Make chia seed pudding by combining chia seeds with unsweetened almond milk and a natural sweetener like stevia or a touch of honey. Top with berries for added sweetness.

Baked Fruit:

- Try baking apples or pears with a sprinkle of cinnamon for a warm and naturally sweet dessert.

Smoothies:

- Prepare smoothies using unsweetened almond milk, a small portion of fruit, spinach or kale, and a scoop of unsweetened protein powder or Greek yogurt. This can satisfy sweet cravings while providing nutrients.

Nut Butter on Whole Grain Bread:

- Spread natural nut butter (like almond or peanut butter) on whole grain toast for a wholesome and slightly sweet snack.

Cinnamon Tea:

- Enjoy a cup of cinnamon tea or herbal teas with natural sweet undertones for a warm, soothing treat.

Smoothie Recipes

Berry Blast Smoothie

Ingredients:

- A cup of berries, comprising strawberries, blueberries, and also raspberries
- 1/2 banana (frozen or fresh)
- 1/2 cup unsweetened Greek yogurt
- 1/2 cup unsweetened almond milk
- Handful of spinach
- Chia seeds (optional)

Instructions:

- Blend mixed berries, banana, Greek yogurt, almond milk, and spinach until smooth.
- Add chia seeds if desired and blend briefly.
- Pour into a glass and enjoy this antioxidant-rich smoothie.

Green Power Smoothie

Ingredients:

- 1 cup spinach

- 1/2 avocado

- 1/2 cup pineapple (fresh or frozen)

- 1/2 cup cucumber

- 1 tablespoon chia seeds

- 1 cup unsweetened coconut water

Instructions:

- Combine spinach, avocado, pineapple, cucumber, and chia seeds in a blender.

- Pour in coconut water and blend until smooth.

- Serve for a nutrient-dense, refreshing green smoothie.

Tropical Paradise Smoothie

Ingredients:

- 1/2 cup mango (fresh or frozen)

- 1/2 banana

- 1/2 cup pineapple

- 1/2 cup unsweetened Greek yogurt

- 1/2 cup unsweetened almond milk

- Handful of spinach (optional)

Instructions:

- Blend mango, banana, pineapple, Greek yogurt, almond milk, and spinach until smooth.
- If necessary, add more almond milk to thin it up.
- Enjoy this tropical-flavored smoothie as a snack or light meal.

Peanut Butter Banana Protein Smoothie

Ingredients:

- 1 ripe banana
- 2 tablespoons natural peanut butter
- 1 scoop unsweetened protein powder (vanilla or unflavored)
- 1 cup unsweetened almond milk
- Handful of ice cubes

Instructions:

- Blend banana, peanut butter, protein powder, almond milk, and ice cubes until creamy.
- Add more almond milk for desired consistency.
- Pour into a glass and relish this protein-rich smoothie.

Chocolate Avocado Smoothie

Ingredients:

- 1/2 avocado

- 1 tablespoon unsweetened cocoa powder

- 1 tablespoon chia seeds

- 1 cup unsweetened almond milk

- Handful of ice cubes

Instructions:

- Blend avocado, cocoa powder, chia seeds, almond milk, and ice cubes until well combined.

- Add more almond milk for a smoother texture, if desired.

- Indulge in this creamy, chocolate-flavored smoothie.

BONUS

30 Day Meal Plan

Day 1

Breakfast: Greek yogurt with mixed berries and chia seeds

Lunch: Grilled chicken salad with mixed greens and balsamic vinaigrette

Dinner: Baked salmon and steamed broccoli and quinoa

Day 2

Breakfast: Spinach and feta omelette

Lunch: Tuna lettuce wraps with avocado slices

Dinner: Stir-fried turkey and vegetables with brown rice

Day 3

Breakfast: Chia seed pudding with sliced strawberries

Lunch: Quinoa salad with grilled shrimp and mixed vegetables

Dinner: Baked tofu with roasted asparagus and a side of sweet potatoes

Day 4

Breakfast: Mixed berry and spinach smoothie

Lunch: Lentil and vegetable soup

Dinner: Grilled lemon herb chicken with roasted bell peppers and cauliflower

Day 5

Breakfast: Almond butter and banana protein smoothie

Lunch: Greek salad with grilled chicken

Dinner: Cod fillet with sautéed zucchini and brown rice

Day 6

Breakfast: Green smoothie with spinach, pineapple, and Greek yogurt

Lunch: Turkey lettuce wraps with mixed vegetables

Dinner: Baked salmon with quinoa and roasted Brussels sprouts

Day 7

Breakfast: Greek yogurt with sliced peaches and almonds

Lunch: Veggie and tofu stir-fry with brown rice

Dinner: Grilled chicken with steamed broccoli and sweet potato

Day 8

Breakfast: Chia seed pudding with mixed berries

Lunch: Mixed greens salad with grilled shrimp

Dinner: Baked tofu with asparagus and quinoa

Day 9

Breakfast: Blueberry and almond butter protein smoothie

Lunch: Lentil soup with mixed green salad

Dinner: Cod fillet with roasted vegetables and brown rice

Day 10

Breakfast: Avocado and tomato on whole-grain toast

Lunch: Greek salad with grilled chicken

Turkey meatballs with zucchini noodles and marinara sauce for dinner

Day 11

Breakfast: Spinach and feta omelette

Lunch: Tuna salad with mixed greens and olive oil vinaigrette

Dinner: Baked chicken breast with roasted veggies and quinoa

Day 12

Breakfast: Greek yogurt with sliced strawberries and chia seeds

Lunch: Turkey lettuce wraps with avocado slices

Dinner: Baked salmon with steamed broccoli and brown rice

Day 13

Breakfast: Blueberry and almond butter smoothie

Lunch: Lentil and vegetable soup

Dinner: Grilled lemon herb chicken with roasted bell peppers and cauliflower

Day 14

Breakfast: Chia seed pudding with mixed berries

Lunch: Quinoa salad with grilled shrimp and mixed vegetables

Dinner: Baked tofu with roasted asparagus and a side of sweet potatoes

Day 15

Breakfast: Almond butter and banana protein smoothie

Lunch: Greek salad with grilled chicken

Dinner: Cod fillet with sautéed zucchini and brown rice

Day 16

Breakfast: Mixed berry and spinach smoothie

Lunch: Veggie and tofu stir-fry with brown rice

Dinner: Baked salmon with quinoa and roasted Brussels sprouts

Day 17

Breakfast: Greek yogurt with sliced peaches and almonds

Lunch: Turkey lettuce wraps with mixed vegetables

Dinner: Grilled chicken with steamed broccoli and sweet potato

Day 18

Breakfast: Chia seed pudding with mixed berries

Lunch: Mixed greens salad with grilled shrimp

Dinner: Baked tofu with asparagus and quinoa

Day 19

Breakfast: Avocado and tomato on whole-grain toast

Lunch: Tuna lettuce wraps with avocado slices

Dinner: Baked chicken breast with roasted veggies and quinoa

Day 20

Breakfast: Green smoothie with spinach, pineapple, and Greek yogurt

Lunch: Lentil soup with mixed green salad

Dinner: Turkey meatballs with zucchini noodles and marinara sauce

Day 21

Breakfast: Greek yogurt with sliced strawberries and almonds

Lunch: Grilled chicken salad with mixed greens and olive oil vinaigrette

Dinner: Baked salmon with steamed broccoli and quinoa

Day 22

Breakfast: Chia seed pudding with mixed berries

Lunch: Quinoa salad with grilled shrimp and mixed vegetables

Dinner: Baked tofu with roasted asparagus and sweet potatoes

Day 23

Breakfast: Blueberry and almond butter smoothie

Lunch: Turkey lettuce wraps with avocado slices

Dinner: Cod fillet with sautéed zucchini and brown rice

Day 24

Breakfast: Mixed berry and spinach smoothie

Lunch: Veggie and tofu stir-fry with brown rice

Dinner: Baked salmon with quinoa and roasted Brussels sprouts

Day 25

Breakfast: Greek yogurt with sliced peaches and chia seeds

Lunch: Mixed greens salad with grilled shrimp

Dinner: Grilled chicken with steamed broccoli and sweet potatoes

Day 26

Breakfast: Green smoothie with spinach, pineapple, and Greek yogurt

Lunch: Tuna salad with mixed greens and olive oil vinaigrette

Dinner: Baked chicken breast with roasted veggies and quinoa

Day 27

Breakfast: Chia seed pudding with mixed berries

Lunch: Turkey lettuce wraps with mixed vegetables

Dinner: Grilled salmon with steamed asparagus and brown rice

Day 28

Breakfast: Almond butter and banana protein smoothie

Lunch: Lentil and vegetable soup

Dinner: Grilled lemon herb chicken with roasted bell peppers and cauliflower

Day 29

Breakfast: Avocado and tomato on whole-grain toast

Lunch: Greek salad with grilled chicken

Dinner: Cod fillet with roasted vegetables and quinoa

Day 30

Breakfast: Greek yogurt with sliced strawberries and almonds

Lunch: Quinoa salad with grilled shrimp and mixed vegetables

Dinner: Baked tofu with roasted asparagus and sweet potatoes

Troubleshooting common challenges

Challenge 1: Sugar Cravings

Tip: Opt for natural sweeteners found in fruits, such as berries or apples, and incorporate healthy fats and proteins in your meals to help curb cravings. Additionally, gradually reduce sugar intake, allowing your taste buds to adjust.

Challenge 2: Portion Control

Tip: Use smaller plates to keep portion quantities under control. Also, focus on nutrient-dense foods that keep you fuller for longer periods, like high-fiber vegetables and lean proteins. Practicing mindful eating and being attentive to hunger cues can also aid in portion control.

Challenge 3: Eating Out and Social Situations

Tip: Plan ahead when dining out by checking the menu in advance and choosing healthier options. Ask for dressings or sauces on the side and opt for grilled or steamed dishes. In social situations, communicate your dietary needs politely and consider bringing a dish that aligns with your diet.

Challenge 4: Lack of Time for Meal Preparation

Tip: Batch cooking and meal prepping can save time during busy weeks. Plan meals in advance, cook in larger quantities, and store portions for easy access. Prepare simple and quick recipes, and use tools like slow cookers or pressure cookers for efficient cooking.

Challenge 5: Stress Eating

Tip: Find alternative stress-relief techniques like meditation, exercise, or hobbies to manage stress. When feeling stressed, opt for healthy snacks like nuts, yogurt, or fresh fruits rather than high-sugar or processed options.

Challenge 6: Plateau in Weight Loss

Tip: Re-evaluate your eating habits and exercise routine. Focus on the quality of the foods you consume, monitor portion sizes, and consider incorporating more physical activity or changing up your workout routine. Sometimes, the body gets accustomed to a certain routine, so introducing variations might help break through a plateau.

Challenge 7: Cravings for Unhealthy Foods

Tip: Understand that occasional indulgences are normal. Instead of depriving yourself entirely, consider healthier alternatives for the foods you crave. Moderation is key; allow yourself a small portion occasionally to satisfy cravings without derailing your progress.

Challenge 8: Consistency and Motivation

Tip: Create a support system, whether it's a friend, family member, or online community, to share experiences and stay motivated. Set achievable short-term goals and celebrate small victories to stay motivated on your journey.

Made in United States
Orlando, FL
10 February 2024

43555944R00039